GENTLE YOGA
BACK PAIN

Featuring Contributions By

LAURIE SANFORD

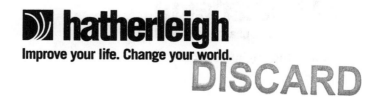

hatherleigh
Improve your life. Change your world.

Gentle Yoga for Back Pain

Text copyright © 2012 Hatherleigh Press

Hatherleigh Press is committed to preserving and protecting the natural resources of the Earth. Environmentally responsible and sustainable practices are embraced within the company's mission statement. Hatherleigh Press is a member of the Publishers Earth Alliance, committed to preserving and protecting the natural resources of the planet while developing a sustainable business model for the book publishing industry.

This book was edited and designed in the village of Hobart, New York. Hobart is a community that has embraced books and publishing as a component of its livelihood. There are several unique bookstores in the village. For more information, please visit www.hobartbookvillage.com.

Library of Congress Cataloging-in-Publication Data is available.
ISBN: 978-1-57826-390-5

Disclaimer
Consult your physician before beginning any exercise program. The author and publisher of this book and workout disclaim any liability, personal or professional, resulting from the misapplication of any of the following procedures described in this publication.

All Hatherleigh Press titles are available for bulk purchase, special promotions, and premiums. For information about reselling and special purchase opportunities, please call 1-800-528-2550 and ask for the Special Sales Manager.

Cover Design by Heather Daugherty
Interior Design by Heather White
Photography by Catarina Astrom

10 9 8 7 6 5 4 3 2 1

Printed in the United States

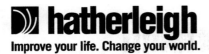

Improve your life. Change your world.

www.hatherleighpress.com

TABLE OF CONTENTS

ACKNOWLEDGMENTS

Hatherleigh Press would like to extend a special thank you to Jo Brielyn—without your hard work and dedication this book would not have been possible.

CHAPTER 1

WHAT IS BACK PAIN?

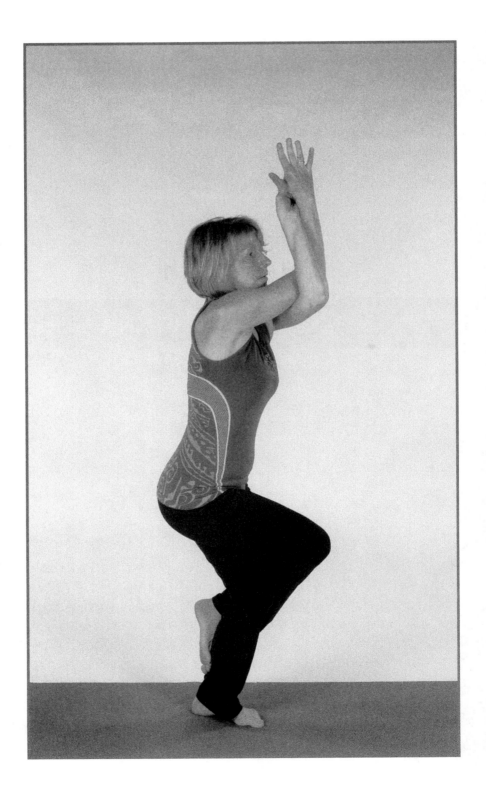

The average person is born with 33 vertebrae (or bones) that connect with each other to make up the vertebral column. By the time most people reach adulthood, they have only 24 vertebrae because the smaller bones at the base of the spine fuse together during development.

The human spine is classified into three main sections: the cervical spine or neck (vertebrae C1-C7), the thoracic spine or mid-back (vertebrae T1-T12), and the lumbar spine or low back (vertebrae L1-L5). At the base of the spine sits a large, triangular bone called the sacrum that is wedged between the two hip bones. The upper part of the sacrum connects with the last lumbar vertebra and the bottom part joins with the coccyx (tailbone).

Joints are positioned on the backside of the vertebrae to enable movement and flexibility in the back. Intervertebral discs sit in between the vertebrae and function like shock absorbers for the spine as it moves. Muscles, ligaments, tendons, and blood vessels are also located in the back. Muscles are threads of tissues that act as the source of power for movement. Ligaments are tough, flexible bands of fibrous tissue that join the bones together, and tendons link muscles to the bones and discs. The blood vessels deliver nourishment to the area. All of these body parts work together to make the back work properly.

Causes of Back Pain

Back pain may be a result of injury to any or all of these parts of the body. Injury to the muscles, tendons, and ligaments can cause sprains or strains, which are generally not serious back issues. However, damage to the bones, intervertebral discs, nerves, or blood vessels in the back may be more serious. Injuries such as ruptured or bulging discs can cause pain and inflammation. Accidents, falls, and bone fractures can result in back pain as well.

Some conditions and diseases may also precipitate back pain, such as:

- Osteoporosis
- Endometriosis
- Fibromyalgia
- Arthritis
- Scoliosis
- Kidney stones
- Spinal stenosis
- Pregnancy
- Infections
- Tumors
- Stress

Back pain is a commonplace physical issue in modern society. In fact, it is currently the most common reason why people in the United States seek medical care. The American Association of Neurological Surgeons reports that over 65 million Americans suffer from back pain each year. Estimates also show that about 80% of Americans will be affected by back pain at some point in their lives.

The term "back pain" encompasses a wide range of symptoms from a dull, constant throbbing to sharp pain that makes it difficult to move and can sometimes be incapacitating. Back pain also comes in many forms, such as lower back pain, middle back pain, upper back pain, and low back pain with sciatica.

Did You Know?
• You are taller in the morning than at night because the discs in your back temporarily compress.
• Americans spend over $50 billion annually on back pain, and that figure only covers the more easily identified costs.
• It is estimated that about 80% (that's 4 out of 5) of adults will experience back pain at some point in their lives.
• Your spine has more than 120 individual muscles, 220 specialized ligaments, and over 100 joints! That means back pain can happen in any of those areas as well as in the discs.
• Most cases of back pain develop in the lower back or lumbar region.
• Back pain is one of the most common reasons cited for missing work.
• Surgery is only necessary in about 2% of cases of back pain.

Common symptoms of back pain include:
• Muscle aches
• Inability to stand straight without having severe muscle spasms in the low back
• Stabbing or shooting pain, usually localized in the neck, upper back, or lower back
• Limited range of motion or flexibility in the back
• Persistent throbbing or stiffness anywhere along the spine, from the base of the neck to the hips
• Chronic aches in the middle or lower back, especially after sitting or standing for extended periods

Common sciatica symptoms:
Sciatica is a common type of back pain that affects the sciatic nerve, which is the large nerve extending from the lower back down the back of each leg. The symptoms of sciatica are different from regular back pain and include:
• Shooting pain that makes it hard to stand up
• Burning or tingling that radiates down the leg

• Pain in the rear or leg that gets worse when you sit
• Weakness, numbness, or difficulty moving the leg or foot
• Constant pain on one side of the rear

You can contact these national organizations to learn more about back pain, ask specific questions, or receive additional information:

American Academy of Orthopaedic Surgeons (AAOS)
Toll-free phone number: (800) 824-BONE / (800) 824-2663
Website: www.aaos.org

American Chiropractic Association
Toll-free phone number: (703) 276-8800
Website: www.acatoday.org

National Institute of Arthritis and Musculoskeletal and Skin Diseases Information Clearinghouse
Toll-free phone number: (877) 22-NIAMS / (877) 226-4267
Website: www.niams.nih.gov

National Institute of Neurological Disorders and Stroke
Toll-free phone number: (800) 352-9424
Website: www.ninds.nih.gov

North American Spine Society (NASS)
Toll-free phone number: (866) 960-NASS / (866) 960-6277
Website: www.spine.org

Risk Factors for Back Pain

Lifestyle factors that increase the risk of developing back pain:

Smoking: In addition to the harmful effects that cigarettes have on the heart and lungs, smoking cigarettes also lowers bone density and increases the risk of fractures.

Sedentary work or inactivity: Sitting for extended periods every day without moving around and lack of regular exercise increase the risk for incidences of lower back pain and increase the probable severity of the pain.

Obesity: Obesity adds more stress on the lower back. The American Academy of Orthopedic Surgeons reports that being overweight increases the risk for developing back pain, and more specifically increases the risk of developing herniated discs.

Poor posture: Prolonged poor posture (such as slouching over a computer, hunching over the steering wheel while driving, and lifting improperly) will greatly increase the risk of developing back pain.

Other risk factors:

Family history: A family history of degenerative spinal conditions such as stenosis, arthritis, and degenerative disc disease put individuals at a higher risk for developing back pain.

Aging: People of any age can experience back pain, but the risk increases with age. Over time, stress on the spine may result in conditions that cause neck and back pain. People between the ages of 30 and 60 are more likely to have disc-related disorders, while people over 60 are more likely to have pain associated with osteoarthritis.

Workplace factors: Doing a job that requires repetitive bending and lifting (such as construction work or nursing) increases the risk of back injury. Occupations that require long hours of standing without a break (such a barber or cashier) also put an individual at a greater risk.

Stress, anxiety, and depression: Psychological and emotional strains often manifest themselves in a physical form in the body. Stress, anxiety, and depression can lead to an increase in muscle cramping and tension. Over time, this strain may also lead to overstretched ligaments and misaligned vertebrae.

Pregnancy: Women who are pregnant may experience more back pain due to the loosening of ligaments in the pelvic area in preparation for delivery, as well as an increase in excess body weight in the abdominal area.

Preexisting medical conditions: Risk of back pain is higher for people who have medical conditions such as osteoporosis, endometriosis, fibromyalgia, arthritis, scoliosis, and spinal stenosis.

Warning Signs That You Should
See a Doctor for Your Back Pain

The majority of back pain improves with time and home treatment. The pain may take weeks to disappear but, in most cases, improvement will be noticeable within the first few days of self-care. If you do not notice improvement or experience an increase in pain, a visit to your doctor is in order.

In rare instances, back pain can also be a warning of a more serious illness. See your doctor if you experience back pain that:

• Is accompanied by inexplicable weight loss
• Occurs after a fall, significant blow to your back, or any other injury
• Causes tingling, numbness, or weakness in one or both of your legs
• Is continual or extreme, especially when you lie down
• Causes new problems with your bladder or bowels
• Increases when you bend forward at the waist or cough
• Is accompanied by a fever
• Extends down one or both legs, particularly if the pain spreads below your knee
• Is associated with pain or pulsing in your abdomen

It is advisable to also speak to your doctor if you begin experiencing back pain for the first time and you are over the age of 50, or if you have a history of steroid use, drug or alcohol abuse, cancer, or osteoporosis.

Common Treatments for Back Pain

Back pain can be acute or chronic. Acute back pain, meaning pain that lasts from a few days to a few weeks, is the culprit of most back pain. It comes on fast and often leaves just as quickly. Acute back pain is generally caused by falling or lifting something heavy and generally goes away without any treatment, although mild pain medications like acetaminophen or ibuprofen may help ease the pain. To be considered acute, the pain should last no longer than 6 weeks.

Chronic pain, on the other hand, can originate quickly or slowly, but persists for longer than three months. Chronic back pain is less common than acute pain and often requires further treatment.

The following are common methods used to relieve the effects of chronic back pain:

Use hot or cold packs. Both hot and cold packs are used to treat pain, depending on the source of the problem. Applying cold will help reduce swelling and help numb deep back pain. Heat works best to ease muscle spasms and pain. The use of hot and cold packs may temporarily help alleviate pain, but this type of treatment does not correct the chronic back pain.

Change behaviors to put less stress on the back. Learning how to properly lift, pull, and push items can lessen the strain placed on your back. Making adjustments to sleep, diet, relaxation, and exercise habits can help, too.

Participate in gentle forms of exercise that relieve stress and build coordination and flexibility. Yoga, some forms of aquatic exercise, and Pilates work well to do this and may also help reduce pain. Some gentle yoga poses may help diminish low back pain by improving strength, balance, and flexibility. Yoga is also helpful for stress reduction and dealing with the psychological aspects of chronic pain.

Consult with a doctor about medications that may help. If the pain is severe enough, your doctor may prescribe medication stronger than ibuprofen or acetaminophen to help. Topical analgesics that come in the form of creams and ointments can be rubbed on the pain site. Anti-inflammatory drugs, muscle relaxers, and injections are also options that a physician may recommend.

Alternative methods are also available. Some individuals seek alternative methods such as chiropractic adjustments, acupressure, and acupuncture to alleviate chronic back pain. It is important to note, though, that some issues may be intensified by some of these methods if the true source of the chronic pain is not clearly identified.

Surgery may be necessary for the most severe cases. The majority of people who suffer with chronic back pain do not need surgery. Surgery is usually only used if all other treatments are ineffective. Instances like herniated discs, spinal stenosis, spondylolisthesis (a condition that causes the vertebrae to slip), vertebral fractures, degenerative disc disease, or spinal tumors may require surgery.

Vitamins and Minerals That Are Beneficial to Your Back

There are a variety of vitamins and minerals that are beneficial for back and bone health and can also help manage pre-existing back pain.

Calcium and vitamin D are the two most essential nutrients that aid in the development, health, and strength of bones. Receiving the daily requirements for these nutrients is especially important for people who have back pain or are at high risk of developing it. Here's why:

Vitamin D is essential for back and bone health because it aids the body in properly using calcium. Vitamin D is important for strong bones, and the body uses it when it creates new bone cells. A deficiency of vitamin D can lead to softening of the bone surfaces, which generally leads to lower back pain. If your body does not get enough vitamin D or it does not absorb it well, you are at greater risk for osteoporosis and bone loss. Increasing vitamin D in the diet significantly improves the condition for people who have chronic lower back pain. Studies also indicate that regular vitamin D intake may lessen the spasms in your lower back. The recommended daily intake of vitamin D is 400 IU (International Units) for infants,; 600 IU for children teenagers, and adults under the age of 50; and 800-1,000 IU for adults 50 and older.

Calcium is a mineral that is vital for building and maintaining strong, healthy bones. Your body stores close to 99% of its calcium in your bones. Children and young adults need adequate calcium intake in order to maximize the amount of calcium stored in their bones. Adults need to get the proper amount of calcium to minimize the loss of calcium stored in their bones. The recommended daily intake of calcium is 1,000 milligrams for children; 1,300 milligrams for teens; 1,000 milligrams for adults under 50; and 1,200 milligrams for adults over the age of 50.

Vitamins A, B12, C, E, and K are important for a strong back and spine, too. Other nutrients like potassium, copper, and magnesium are also beneficial. Below are some natural ways to get more of these important vitamins and nutrients to boost and maintain the health of your bones and back:

Natural Sources of Calcium:
• Milk
• Cheese
• Plain low-fat yogurt
• Sardines
• Salmon
• Any seafood that contains bones
• Turnip greens
• Spinach
• Kale
• Broccoli

• Nuts (almonds, Brazil nuts, and pecans)
• Legumes (peas, lentils, and beans)

Natural Sources of Vitamin D:
• Sunlight
• Dairy products
• Eggs
• Milk
• Tuna
• Liver oils
• Mackerel
• Cod
• Sea bass

Natural Sources of Vitamin A:
• Dairy products
• Milk
• Eggs
• Yellow vegetables (summer squash)
• Carrots
• Liver
• Green leafy vegetables (kale, spinach, greens, and romaine lettuce)
• Fruits (cantaloupe, tomatoes, and apricots)

Natural Sources of Vitamin B12:
• Liver
• Lean beef
• Clams
• Salmon
• Haddock
• Trout
• Cheese
• Dairy
• Eggs

Natural Sources of Vitamin C:
- Citrus
- Papayas
- Green vegetables
- Berries

Natural Sources of Vitamin E:
- Dark green leafy vegetables
- Nuts
- Vegetable oils
- Whole grains
- Wheat germ

Natural Sources of Vitamin K:
- Seeds
- Eggs
- Dairy products
- Broccoli
- Brussels sprouts
- Chickpeas

Natural Sources of Potassium:
- Milk
- Green leafy vegetables (romaine lettuce, spinach, Swiss chard, and greens)
- Broccoli
- Lentils
- Winter squash
- Fruits (tomatoes, cantaloupe, avocado, oranges, and strawberries)
- Snapper
- Halibut
- Scallops
- Soy
- Potatoes (white and sweet varieties)

Natural Sources of Copper:
• Vegetables
• Liver
• Legumes
• Nuts
• Seeds
• Beans

Natural Sources of Magnesium:
• Brazil nuts
• Seeds (sunflower seeds, pumpkin seeds, and sesame seeds)
• Bananas
• Legumes
• Tofu
• Green leafy vegetables (spinach, Swiss chard, and kelp)
• Whole grains (barley, brown rice, and oats)

CHAPTER 2

THE BENEFITS OF YOGA

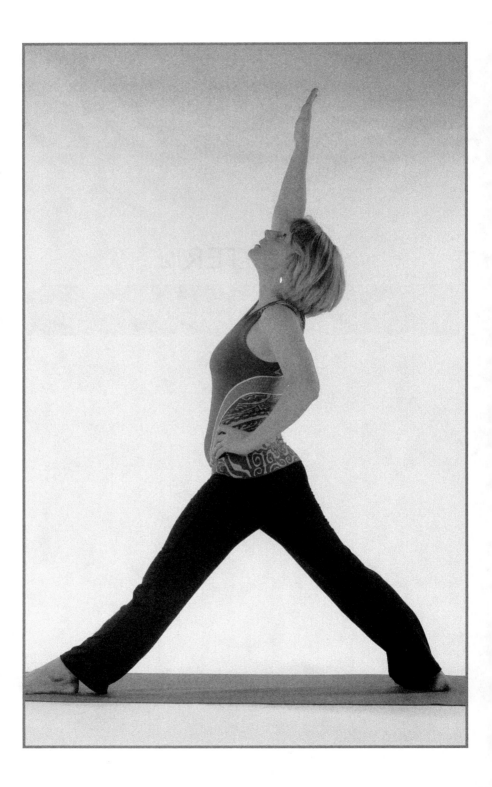

Yoga works well for maintaining health and managing back pain. Those who regularly practice the discipline have known this for ages, but a December 2005 study funded by the National Center for Complementary and Alternative Medicine (NCCAM) at the National Institutes of Health revealed data to back up this claim. The study determined that individuals with chronic lower back pain who regularly participated in a 12-week session of yoga classes experienced less pain and had more improved function than those in the other groups who took conventional exercise classes or practiced home self-care. A 26-week follow-up with the yoga participants found that they also had continued pain relief and function improvement while requiring less pain medication.

Yoga offers many benefits such as relieving pain, stress, and anxiety. It also :

Offers relief from pain, stress and anxiety: Yoga is effective in alleviating pain and reducing stress and anxiety, which can compromise systems in your body and affect functions like immunity and digestion. Yoga practices such as meditation help the individual focus on something other than what he or she feels. It also allows the entire body to relax and get the rest it needs to replenish itself.

Strengthens muscles and increases flexibility: Strong and flexible muscles boost the strength of the bones they surround and offer them added protection. Yoga provides a way to strengthen muscles and build flexibility in the back and abdominal muscles that support the spine. Strengthening your muscles, particularly those in the back and shoulders, also helps improve your posture.

Stretches the muscles: Yoga requires that you hold gentle poses for several seconds to a minute, which helps stretch the muscles gradually over time. Proper stretching of the muscles is important, particularly for those who have lower back pain, because it decreases the stress placed across the lower back.

Promotes good posture: Good posture is important for maintaining a strong, healthy, and flexible spine. Yoga exercises, especially the seated and standing poses, help improve posture and the alignment of the spine. Proper posture relieves some of the pressure off the spine and reduces back pain.

Yoga and the Mind-Body Connection

Yoga is a mind-body kind of exercise that helps you stay fit and relaxed, and is also beneficial for managing chronic back pain. Since yoga combines movement and conscious breathing exercises, it helps you focus both on what your body is physically doing and what is occurring internally. As the root "yuj" (meaning unity or yoke) implies, yoga is an exercise form that seeks to unify the mind and body. When that union takes place, it brings with it a wealth of therapeutic benefits.

The practice of yoga can be traced back to over 5000 years ago, to a time when monks in India (called yogi) secluded themselves and sat for hours in deep meditation in an attempt to create strong, disease-free bodies. While they found the meditation good for the mind, their sore bodies would not allow them to stay in the same position for extended periods. Instead, they had to change positions while still focusing on their meditation. Over time, more structured yoga postures stemmed from these early practices and addressed specific needs in the body as well as the mind.

Today, yoga is used in many therapeutic ways, such as to detoxify, relieve anxiety and depression, realign musculature, strengthen muscles, create flexibility, and manage chronic pain.

"Yoga teaches us to cure what need not be endured, and endure what cannot be cured." —B.K.S. Iyengar

**Learn more about yoga and
its benefits on these websites:**

American Yoga Association
www.americanyogaassociation.org

International Association of Yoga Therapists
www.iayt.org

Yoga Journal
www.yogajournal.com

Meditation Tips for Beginners

Yoga offers meditation and controlled breathing techniques that can be used effectively to manage back pain and refocus your thoughts. Meditating for only a few minutes each day can help.

Here are a few quick tips for meditation beginners:

• Take the time to stretch out first. Loosening muscles and tendons before beginning allows you to sit or lie down more comfortably.

• Make it a formal practice by setting aside a specific time and place to devote to your meditation.

• Focus on your breathing. Slowing your breathing helps your mind and body to relax and prepare for meditation.

• Meditate in the morning. It is usually quieter in the morning, and your mind has not yet had the chance to get cluttered. It will also help work out any kinks in your body from sleeping. And it's always great to start your day with focus!

• Find a time and place to meditate where you will not be disturbed.

• Enlist the help of instructional videos or calming music if they help you relax more.

• Light a candle and use it as a focal point, instead of closing your eyes. Focusing on the light causes you to strengthen your attention.

• Be aware of your body and how it feels in both its normal and relaxed states, and embrace the differences.

• Experiment with different types of meditation and different positions. You won't know which methods work best for you until you try them.

• Have a purpose behind your meditation, such as pain management or feeling more focused on a specific issue you must deal with.

• Push aside any feelings of doubt, frustration, and stress about whether or not you are doing it right. It is counterproductive to your meditation.

• Relax and relish in your mind's incredible ability to focus and care for your body through meditation.

• Remember your meditation and breathing techniques throughout the day. A few well-placed cleansing breaths will do wonders for your mind and body.

Many of the most commonly recommended yoga poses to combat and relieve back pain can be found in this book, including:

Warrior II
Reverse Warrior
Half Moon
Reverse Triangle
Full Squat
Yoga Squat/Forward Bend
Cobra
Fish
Eagle
Camel/Half Camel
Cat and Dog
Recline Big Toe
Locust
Sphinx
Upward-Facing Bent Leg

Did You Know?

• Yoga has been practiced in America since late 19th century but only gained popularity around the 1960s.
• Yoga can relieve pain from many chronic conditions.
• According to the Benson-Henry Institute for Mind-Body Medicine (previously the Mind Body Medical Institute at Harvard Medical School), chronic pain patients who practice meditation reduce their physician visits by 36%.
• Yoga can be practiced virtually anywhere. Variations can even be done at your desk or in your car.
• Yoga and diet go hand in hand. There are foods you can eat that will actually increase your brain function and flexibility.
• A man who practices yoga is called a yogi or yogin. A woman who does is called a yogini.

CHAPTER 3

SAFETY PRECAUTIONS

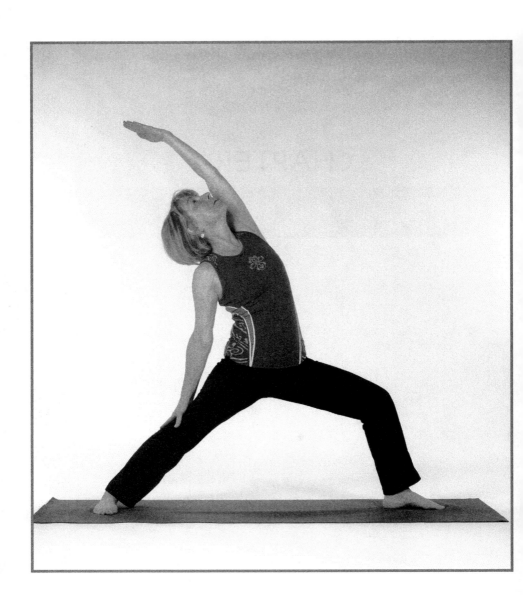

L earning the proper ways to move, sit, and stand can help you stay mobile and active, while also protecting against future back pain. Maintaining good posture helps combat against curvature of the spine. Alignment (which is the way the head, shoulders, spine, hips, knees, and ankles line up with each other) is important for sustaining proper posture. When the body is properly aligned, it also puts less stress on the spine and results in less back pain.

Even though an active lifestyle is healthy, there are some exercises that may actually cause more harm than good. If you have chronic back pain or any past broken bones in the spine, it is best to avoid exercises that involve bending over from the waist (like toe-touches, abdominal crunches, and sit-ups). When you bow forward at the waist, the shoulders and back become rounded and can increase the risk of fracturing the spine or doing more damage to your back.

Some forms of exercise that involve bending and twisting motions can be modified to gain the benefits, while not placing too much stress on the spine. Yoga is one beneficial practice that can be modified safely. It's important to remember that as your body changes and matures, the way you practice yoga must also change. Approach your yoga exercises with gentleness and acceptance of the body you have now, and allow it to work well for you.

Follow these guidelines to ensure safety when practicing yoga exercises for back pain:

• Rule out any serious or potentially life-threatening causes for your back pain (such as cancer, rupturing aortic aneurisms, or infections) before you begin a yoga regimen. While it is less common for these types of issues to be the cause of back pain, it is wise to be sure it is safe for you to begin an exercise program, especially if you are experiencing any troublesome symptoms such as unusual weight loss or fever, or if you are over the age of 50.

• It is always recommended that you talk to your doctor before starting an exercise program. This is especially true if you already have chronic back pain.

• Once you have the approval of your doctor, start the exercise program and ease into the more difficult moves. These gentle yoga exercises are intended to strengthen your body and relieve some of the symptoms associated with your back pain, not aggravate them.

• If you are new to yoga, you may find it best to start by holding the poses for only a few long, deep breaths. As you progress and feel more comfortable, you can begin to hold the poses for longer.

• If you have lumbar disc issues, use extreme caution when doing forward bends and poses that involve a great deal of twisting. Also, be sure to slowly ease into transitions from one pose to the next and try stepping instead of jumping into poses.

• Concentrate more on maintaining proper alignment while doing your yoga exercises, and focus less on pushing over your limits. Recognize your limitations and respect them. Trying to surpass your limits may inflict unnecessary pain or risk of injury.

• Since everyone has varying degrees of flexibility and pain associated with existing back issues, it is important not to gauge your level of difficulty against someone else's. Practice the yoga exercises to the degree that you can perform them comfortably and safely for your own body.

• If any of the yoga moves cause pain in your back, listen to your body and stop immediately.

Yoga Postures to Avoid When Dealing with Back Pain

Forward Bend: The standing forward bend (also known as Uttanasana) should be avoided or modified if you have a problem with your lower back. The pose can be modified by trying to stand with your feet slightly apart. You may also want to enlist the help of yoga props such as a chair or yoga blocks. Simply place your hands on the yoga blocks or seat of the chair, instead of using the floor. If your back pain is severe, you may want to avoid modified versions of forward bends as well.

Headstand: If you have back pain, do not attempt to do a headstand (also known as Sirsasana). This pose requires a great deal of balance and strength, and any weakness in your spine could cause you to do it incorrectly. Performing a headstand improperly could exacerbate an existing back injury or cause a new one.

Reclining Hero Pose: The reclining hero pose (also known as Supta Virasana) is done while sitting between your heels and leaning backwards. This pose should not be performed by anyone with spinal disorders, unless don with the help of yoga props. Instead of placing your upper body flat on the floor, use folded blankets to elevate yourself and make the pose safer. If you have a severe spinal condition, do not try this pose or any modification of it.

Backbend: A backbend might be beneficial for specific types of back problems, but can be dangerous for people who suffer from spondylolisthesis. It is best to use yoga props whenever necessary and exercise extreme caution when performing backbends, even if you do not have severe back problems. If you experience back pain, ask your instructor if there are modifications of this pose that you can do safely with your current back issues.

Practical Tips to Protect Against Back Pain

- Maintain a healthy weight and diet.
- Stay active (under the guidance of your doctor or chiropractor).
- Wear comfortable, low-heeled shoes.
- Avoid long periods of inactivity or bed rest whenever possible.
- Sleep on a mattress of medium firmness to reduce any cur vature in your spine.
- Always stretch or warm up before you exercise or participate in any physical activity.
- Work at an ergonomically correct computer workstation.
- Be aware of maintaining proper posture.
- Practice proper lifting techniques:
    - Spread your feet apart and straddle the object.
    - Stand close to the object to be lifted.
    - Squat, bend your knees and hips, and keep your back in proper alignment.
    - Tighten your stomach muscles.
    - Lift by using your leg muscles, not your back.
    - When lifting with another individual, designate one person to say when to lift, move, and unload.
    - Do not twist while you lift the object. Instead, turn with your hips and shoulders in line and shift your weight.

CHAPTER 4

THE POSES

MOUNTAIN

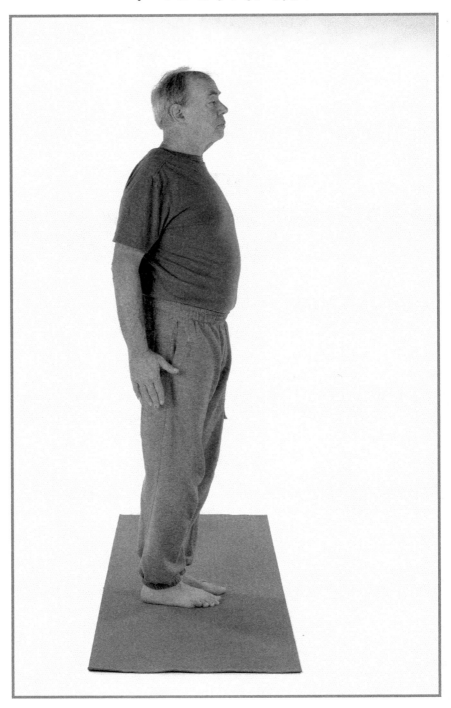

MODIFICATION

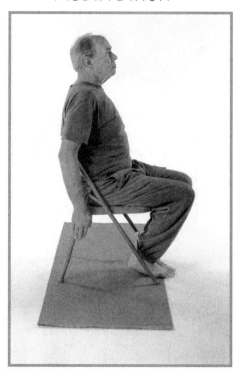

Stand with your big toes touching. Roll your shoulders up, back, and down—this movement places your shoulder blades on your back. Try to find your balance over the arches of your feet by rocking back and forth from the balls of your feet to the heels. Then build your body up from your feet and through your calves, pulling your kneecaps up, tightening your thighs, and tucking your tailbone under. Your chin should be centered with your chest. Exhale and pull up on your pelvic floor. On the next exhale, pull your stomach up and back (this will create strength in your abdominals). This "lock" in the abdominals should be used in all standing postures.

For the chair variation, sit upright in a chair with your legs and feet together and your arms at your sides. Roll your shoulders up, back, and down, then follow the directions to create a "lock" in your abdominals.

WARM-UP FORWARD BEND

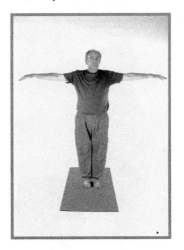

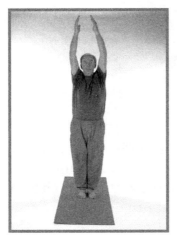

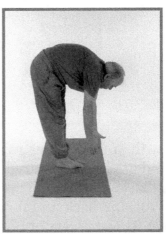

Stand with your feet together in Mountain pose (see page 32). On the inhale, sweep your arms up and over your head. Reach up and then back, stretching through both sides of your torso with your weight in your heels. On the exhale, swan-dive down into a forward bend from the hips, with your arms out to your sides, leading with your chin and chest. Sweep your hands close to the floor and inhale all the way up and back again. Repeat five to six times.

MODIFICATION

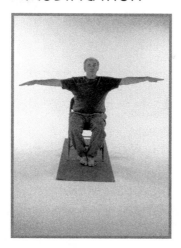

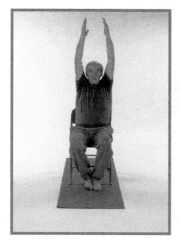

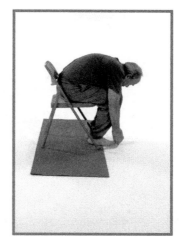

For the chair variation, sit in the chair and face forward with your legs and feet together. Sweep your arms up and then on the exhale, bend down over your legs. On the inhale, come up and reach back. In the beginning, your back may be rounded. As you gain strength, try to come down and up with a straight back.

Note: You should always be aware of any pain or straining in the legs or back and be sure to only do what is comfortable for you

WARRIOR I

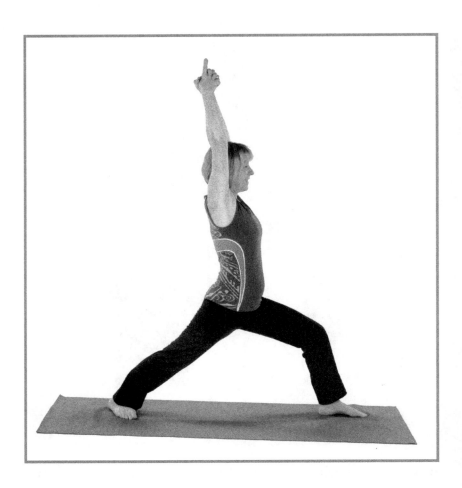

Start with your feet together in Mountain pose (see page 32). Take a wide-legged stance and turn your left foot out 90 degrees. Turn to face over your left foot with your shoulders and your hips. On the exhale, bend your left knee. On the inhale, raise your arms over your head and interlock your fingers. For increased intensity (not pictured), look up at your hands and hold for five breaths. Repeat on the other side.

MODIFICATION

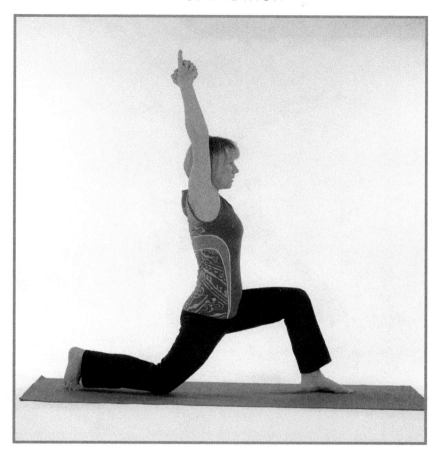

If this seems difficult, you may drop your back knee to the floor until you gain balance and strength.

WARRIOR II

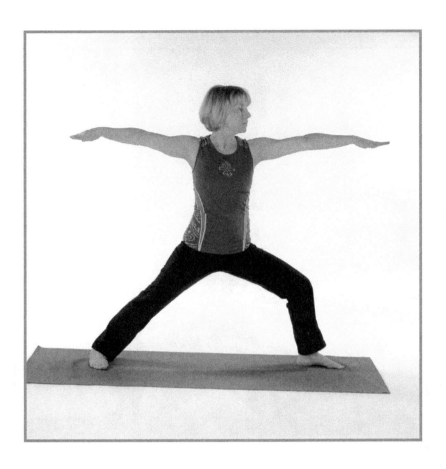

Start with your feet together in Mountain pose (see page 32). Take a wide-legged stance and, on the exhale, turn your left foot out 90 degrees, keeping your hips and shoulders facing forward. On the inhale, raise your arms into a 'T' position. On the next exhale, bend your left knee over your ankle. Your weight should be on the outside of your right foot as you pull up in your inner right thigh. Your focal point will be at the fingertips of your left hand. Hold for five breaths. Repeat on the other side.

MODIFICATION

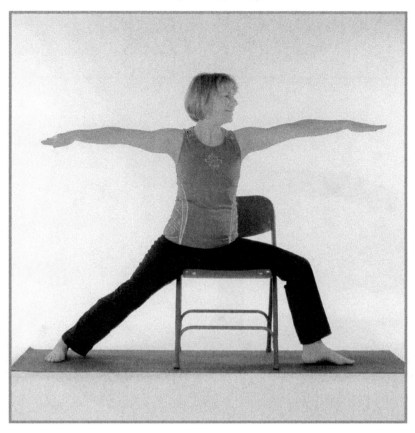

For the chair variation, sit on a chair and come to a straddle position. Bend your left knee and turn your left foot out 90 degrees. Extend your right leg out straight. On the inhale, raise your arms up and hold for five breaths.

WARRIOR III

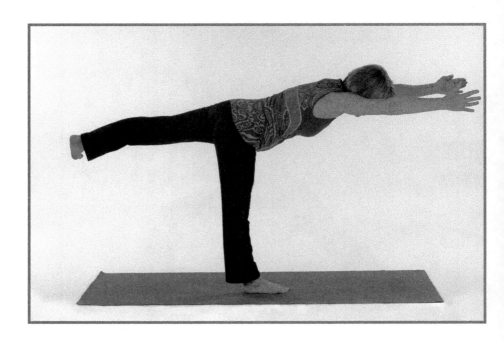

Start with your feet together, placing your weight on your right foot. On the inhale, raise your arms shoulder-width over your head. On the exhale, come forward with your torso and raise your left leg behind, keeping your hips parallel. Tighten your right leg and your abdominal muscles to hold your body up. Work up to five breaths. Repeat on the other side.

MODIFICATION

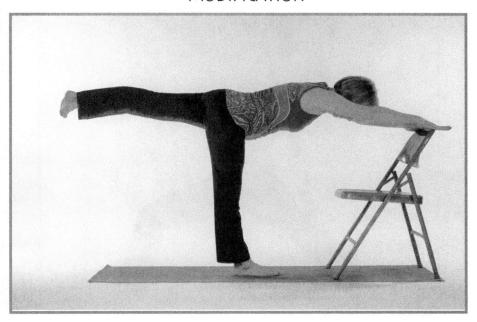

If this seems difficult, the pose can also be performed with your hands against the wall or on a chair, as shown.

Note: Beginners should begin by working with the chair, making sure to bend from the hips.

REVERSE WARRIOR

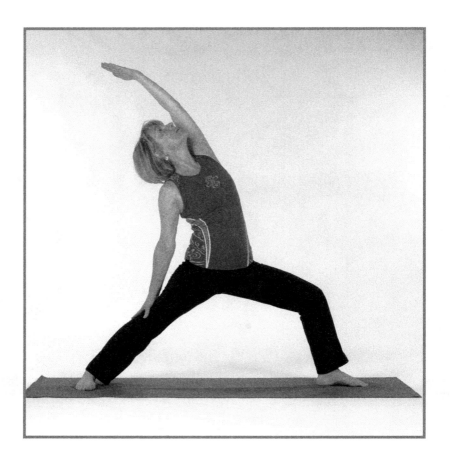

Start in Warrior II pose (see page 38), facing to the left (your legs will not move throughout this sequence). Position your arms out in a 'T' position. On the inhale, drop your right hand down to your right leg as you raise your left arm straight up. Exhale and bend your left arm over your head as you bend your torso back, stretching the left side of your body up and back. Hold for five breaths. Repeat on the other side.

MODIFICATION

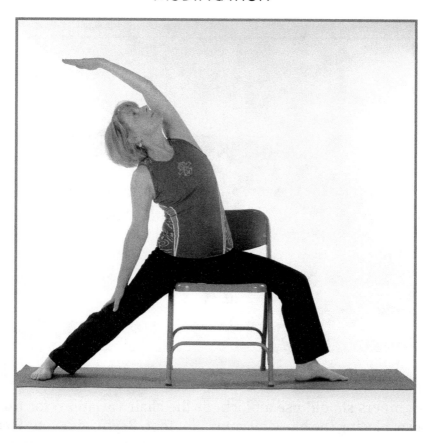

For the chair variation, start by sitting on a chair. Straddle the chair, bending your left knee as you turn your left foot out 90 degrees. Extend your right leg out straight and then follow the arm directions.

Note: When moving into this back and side bend, be aware of the point where you begin to feel any resistance in the body and stop at that point. As you become more flexible, you will be able to move deeper into the pose.

HALF MOON

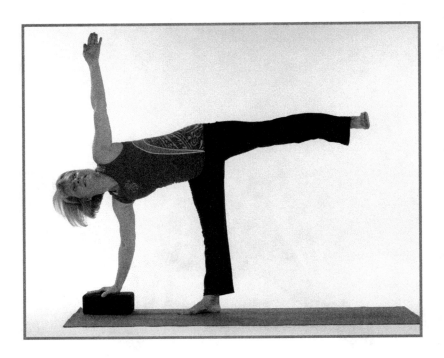

Beginners should use a block (or the chair variation) for this pose, placing the block by your right foot. Begin with your feet together in Mountain pose (see page 32) in the middle of the mat. Take a wide-legged stance, turn your right foot out 90 degrees, and bend your right knee so that your chest is resting on your right thigh. Place the block in your hand and bring it at least six inches in front of your right foot, keeping it in line with your baby toe. On the inhale, straighten your right leg while lifting your left. Keep your weight in your right leg and hand. Tighten your abdominals and both legs (the block has three levels, so start at the highest level and as you gain strength and balance use the lower levels).

MODIFICATION

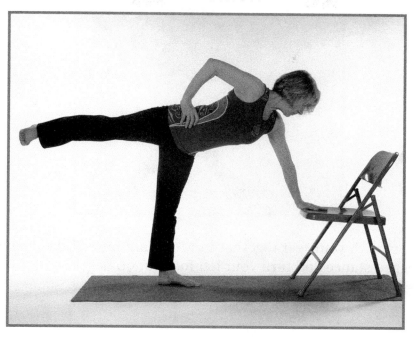

Place your left hand on your waist and work up to five full breaths. As this pose becomes easier, you may wish to increase the intensity by raising your left arm up towards the ceiling while turning your head to look up at your hand. You may also use a different height on the block, working towards the goal of placing your hand on the floor. Repeat on the other side.

For the chair variation, place a chair six to ten inches away from your right foot. In a wide-legged stance, proceed as described above, placing your hand on the chair for balance.

REVERSE TRIANGLE

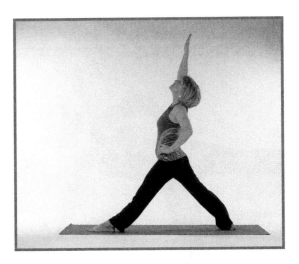

Start with your feet together in Mountain pose. Take a wide-legged stance and turn your left foot out 90 degrees.

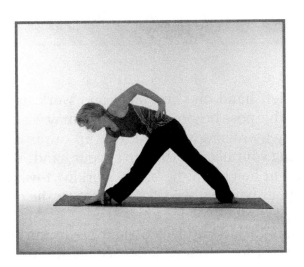

Place the block (if using) on the outside of your left foot and then turn your body to face over your left foot with both hips and shoulders facing left. Place your left hand on your hip.

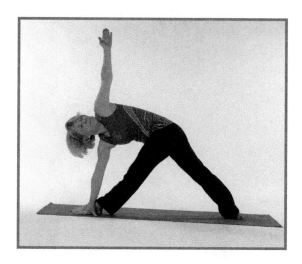

On the inhale, raise your right arm up and back, stretching back. On the exhale, start the twist as you come forward, placing your right hand to your knee, the block, or the floor. Hold for five breaths. For increased intensity, raise your left arm towards the ceiling while looking up at your hand.

When using the block, remember that it has three heights and beginners should start with the highest level.

Note: This pose should be done from the hips, not the waist. As always, use caution and be sure to "listen" to the body—if the pose becomes too difficult, stop or switch to a more gentle variation.

LATERAL STRETCH

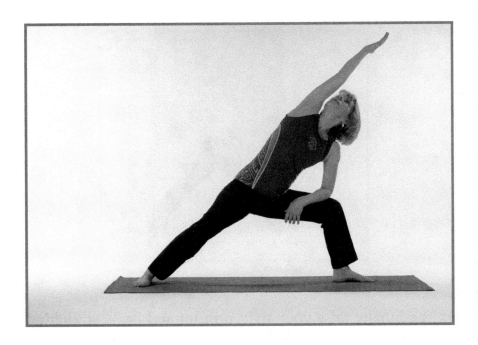

Start with your feet together in Mountain pose (see page 32) in the middle of the mat. Take a wide-legged stance and turn your right foot out 90 degrees. On the exhale, bend your right knee, keeping the outside of your left foot on the floor. On the exhale, drop your right forearm to your thigh and, on the inhale, raise your left arm up. On the next exhale, stretch your left arm over your head while stretching from your left foot through your leg, hips, ribs and out from the fingertips of your left hand. With your palm facing down, turn your head to look at your palm—this keeps your neck in line with your spine. Hold for five breaths and repeat on the left side. As you gain strength in your legs, you may try this by using a block on the outside of your right foot. On the exhale, place your right hand down to the block and proceed as before. This pose may also be done with a chair by straddling the chair, positioning your legs in Warrior II (see page 38) and then proceeding with the arm movements.

FULL SQUAT

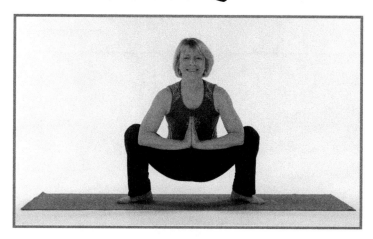

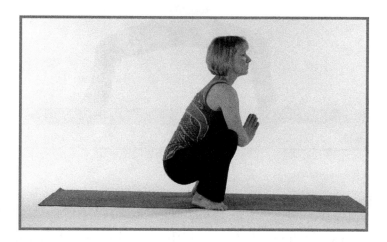

Start with your feet a little more than hip-width apart and your toes pointing out (your feet can be out as far as the edge of the mat). Bring your hands together in prayer position and bend your knees, coming down as far as you can while keeping the soles of your feet on the ground. Work up to five breaths. To come up, place your hands on the floor and straighten your legs, then slowly roll your spine up.

YOGA SQUAT/FORWARD BEND

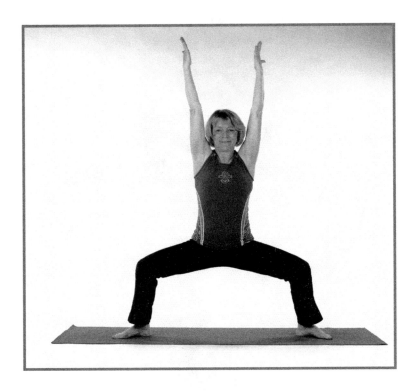

Stand in a wide-legged stance with your feet pointing out. On the inhale, bend your knees and come down halfway while raising your arms into a wide 'V' position.

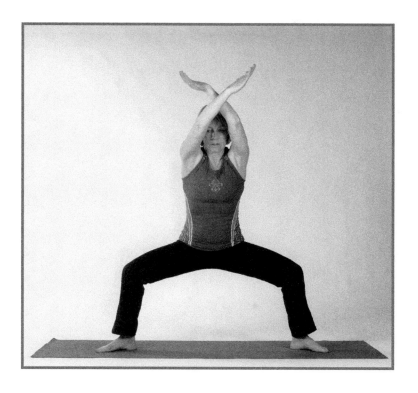

On the exhale, keep your legs where they are and cross your arms above your head.

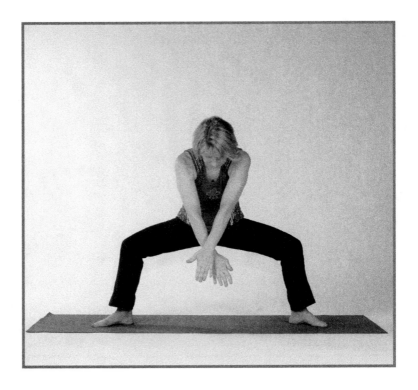

Bend forward halfway, with your arms crossed in front of your body.

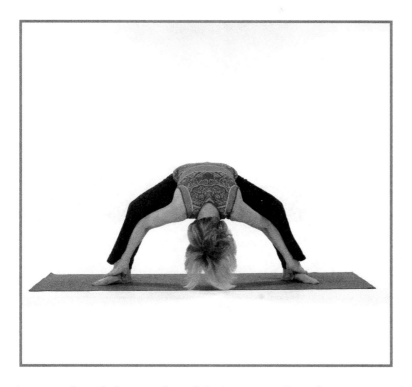

Continue to bend forward and bring your hands to your ankles and your elbows to your knees.

On the next inhale, rise back up into the "V" position. On the exhale, lower down again. Repeat four to five times.

Note: This pose should be done from the hips, not the waist. Once your hands are under your toes, raise your head to keep your spine in alignment and prevent a "hump" in your back.

This pose can also be done with your hands on a chair so that you can straighten your back. As always, use caution and be sure to "listen" to the body—if the pose becomes too difficult, stop or switch to a more gentle variation.

COBRA

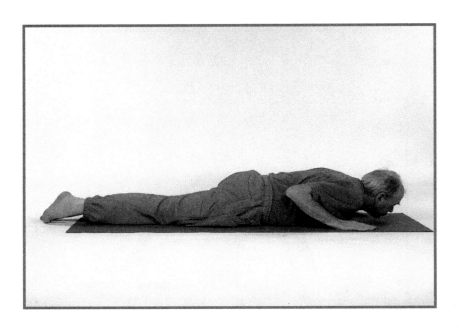

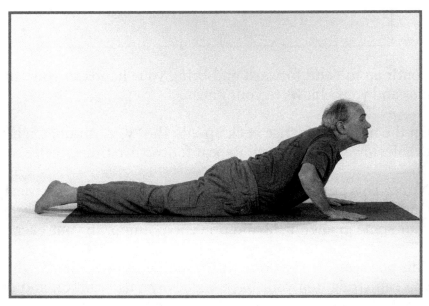

MODIFICATION

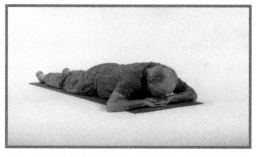

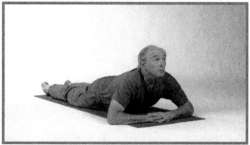

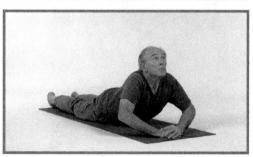

Start by lying on the mat on your stomach. Bring your feet and legs together and keep your forehead to the floor. Bring your hands under your shoulders and on the inhale, push your body up with your arms and roll your shoulders up and back while expanding your chest and keeping your hips on the floor (this will work the lower back). Hold for three full breaths and release down. Come up again and hold for three more full breaths.

Note: As always, use caution and be sure to "listen" to your body—if the pose becomes too difficult, stop or switch to a more gentle variation.

CAMEL/HALF CAMEL

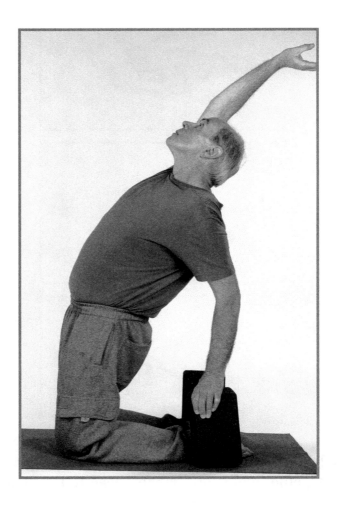

Come onto your knees. Place your hands on your lower back, rocking back as you support your body with your hands. Place a block (start by using the highest level and lower as you become more flexible) next to your left heel, twist, and place your left hand on the block or on your heel. Lean back and extend your right arm behind you as you push your hips forward. Try to work up to four or five breaths. Repeat on the other side.

MODIFICATION

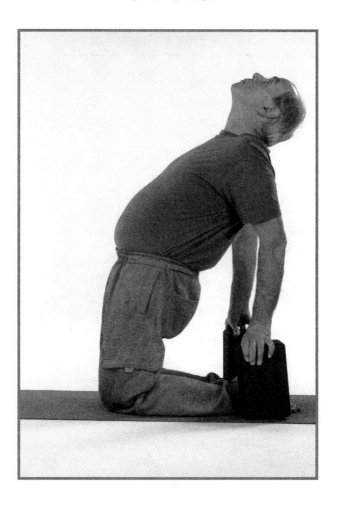

For increased intensity, you can perform the full camel using two blocks or heels, placing your hands on your heels/blocks. Let your head release back towards the floor and push your hips forward.

Note: This pose is a deep back bend and may require you to start by practicing lesser back bends to increase your flexibility with Camel pose as a final goal.

SEATED TWIST

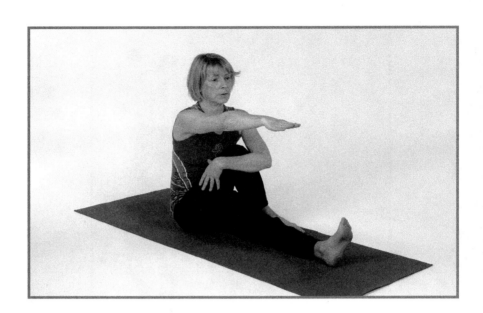

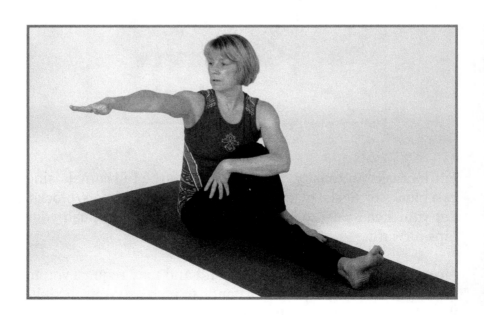

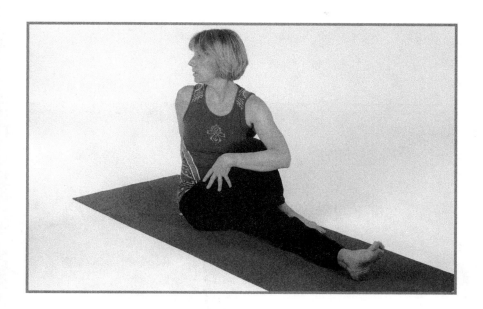

Sit with your legs together and extended straight out. Bring your right leg up and cross it over your left leg, placing the sole of your right foot on the outside of your left thigh. Hold your right knee with your left arm, raising your right arm straight out in front of your body. On the exhale, turn to your right with your arm extended and follow with your head, placing your hand on the floor behind your back. Hold for five breaths and slowly release by first turning your head forward, then releasing your leg. Repeat on the other side.

Note: Be sure to only twist as far as is comfortable, being careful not to twist your neck too far.

RECLINED SPINAL TWIST

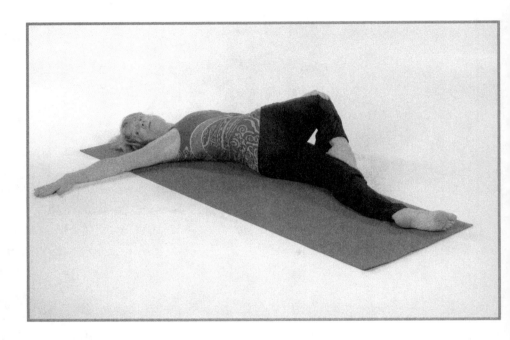

Lie on your back with your legs and feet together. Bring your right foot up and place the sole on your left thigh. Place your right arm out into a 'T' position and position your left hand on the outside of your right knee. On the exhale, twist to the left with your knee and look to the right with your head. Twist until you feel resistance and then hold for five breaths. Repeat on the other side.

MODIFICATION

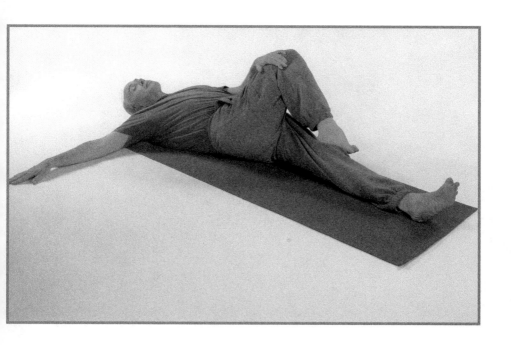

If you are unable to twist all the way to the left, you can twist halfway or as far as is comfortable for you.

BRIDGE

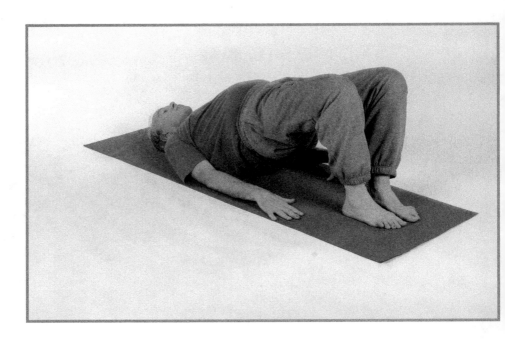

Start on your back with your knees bent. Bring your heels as close to your buttocks as possible. On the inhale, raise your hips up, keeping your legs and feet parallel (you may place a block at a height that is comfortable for you and position it at the top of your buttocks, or use your hands to help hold your body up).

MODIFICATION

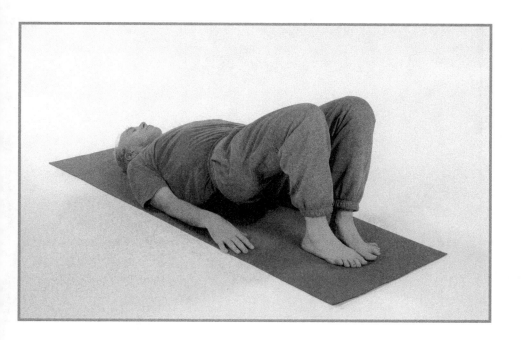

Work up to five full breaths. Once this becomes easy, you can try bringing your hands together under your body and interlock your fingers with your arms straight and your chin to your chest (not pictured). Follow this pose with Fish (see page 64).

If you are unable to lift your hips all the way, you can lift them halfway or as far as is comfortable for you.

FISH

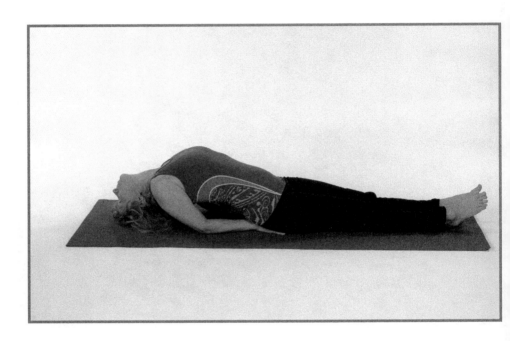

Lie on your back and bring your hands under your buttocks with your palms facing down. On the inhale, raise your upper body onto your elbows. On the exhale, arch your back, trying to place the top of your head on the mat while looking at the wall or floor behind you.

MODIFICATION

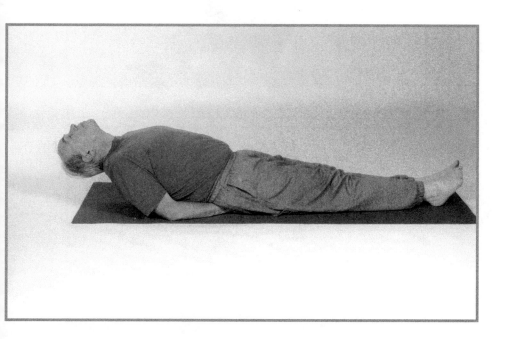

Hold for the same number of breaths that you held for the Bridge pose (this pose should be done after Bridge, page 62, as Bridge creates a constriction in the throat and Fish creates an opening in the throat).

If its is uncomfortable to place the top of your head on the mat, you can keep your head in line with your spine, facing the ceiling above.

BOAT

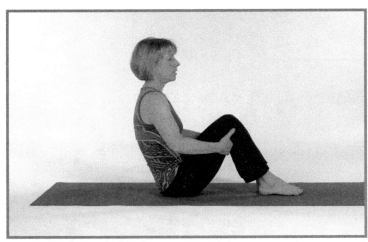

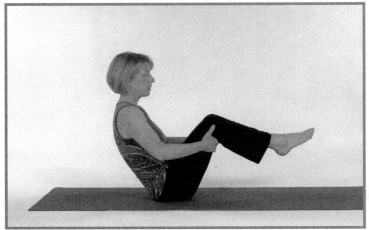

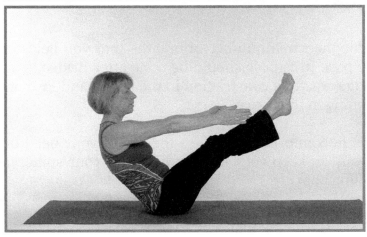

MODIFICATION

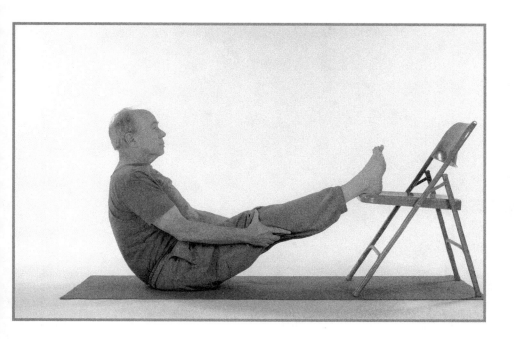

Come to a sitting staff position (sit on the mat with your back straight and your legs out in front of you). Bend your knees and bring the soles of your feet to the floor as you grab behind your knees. Rock back, holding your legs until your feet come off the floor. Try to straighten your legs and hold (you may continue to hold your legs until your abdominal muscles become strong enough to hold your body up). For increased intensity, stretch your arms out along the sides of your legs and hold for five or more breaths.

For the chair variation, place a chair in front of you and bring your feet onto the edge of the chair, proceeding as described above.

EAGLE

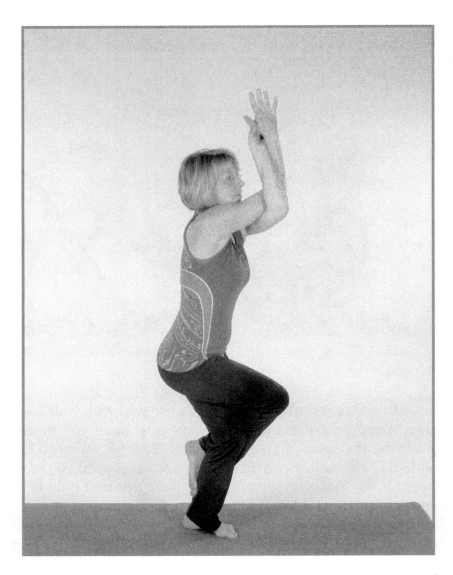

Start with your feet together in Mountain pose (see page 32). Put your weight in your left foot, bring your right arm on top of the left, and intertwine the arms to bring the hands together. Bend your left leg and wrap your right leg around your left as you bring your hands either under your chin or raise them. Hold for 5 breaths.

SPHINX

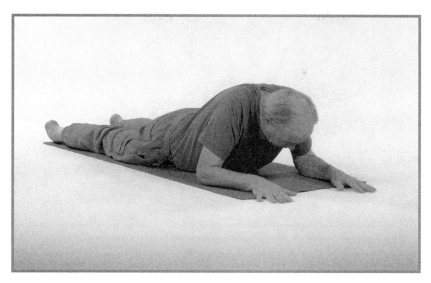

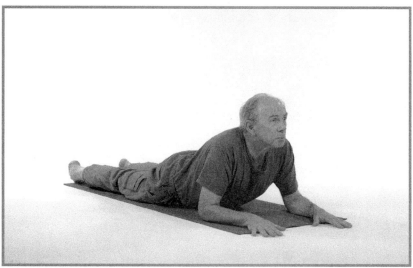

Lie on your stomach and bring your forehead to the floor.
With your legs and feet together, bring your arms up and position your elbows under your shoulders, keeping your fore-
arms stretched out in front of your torso. On the inhale, rise
up onto your elbows and hold for five breaths or more. Come
down, take a breath or two, and then rise back up for another
five breaths.

RECLINE BIG TOE

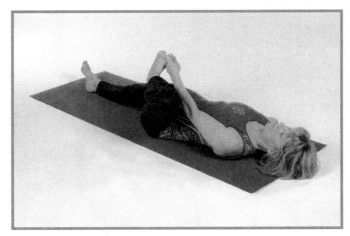

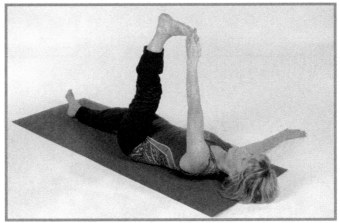

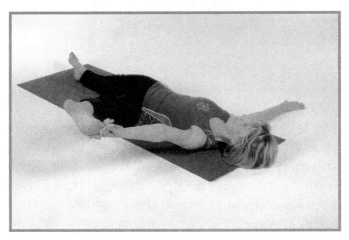

MODIFICATION

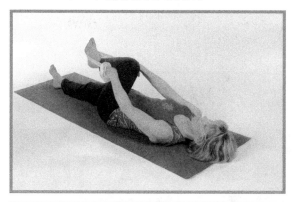

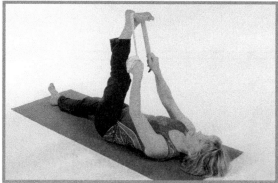

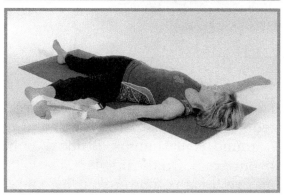

Lie on your back on the mat with your legs and feet together. Bend your left knee and grab your big toe with your thumb and forefinger (if this is too difficult, you may use a strap, as shown, and wrap it around your foot). Straighten your leg up-ward and with your right arm out in a 'T' position, try bringing your left leg out to the left. Hold and repeat on the other side.

LOCUST

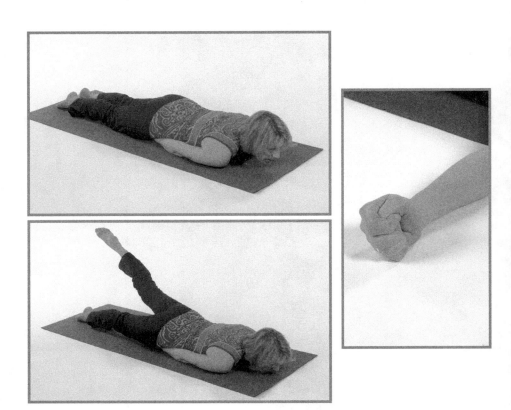

Lie on your stomach with your chin on the floor and your legs and feet together. Make a fist with your hand by wrapping your fingers around your thumbs. Bring your hands under your body at your groin. On the inhale, raise your left leg and hold for up to five breaths. Lower your leg and, on the next inhale, raise your right leg and hold, keeping your chin on the floor.

Variation 1 (not pictured): Bring your hands under your body with your palms down and pinkies touching. Repeat the sequence.

MODIFICATION

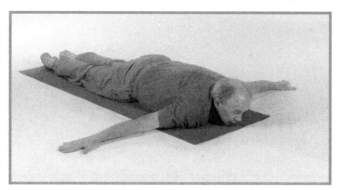

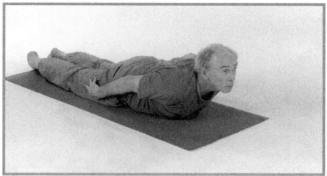

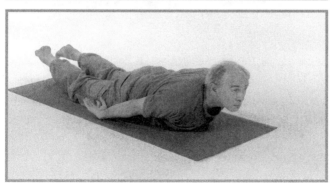

Variation 2: Bring your arms out in a 'T' position and, on the inhale, sweep them back and raise your head and chest. Raise your legs.

MODIFICATION

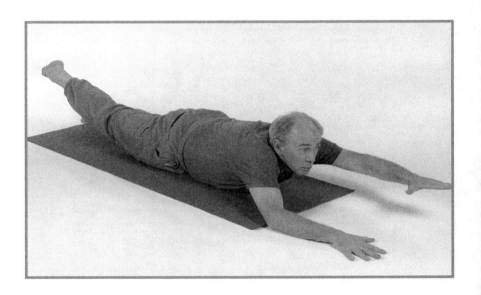

Variation 3: Bring your arms out in front of your body and raise your left arm and right leg, hold, then lower. Raise your right arm and left leg, hold, then lower. Finally, raise both arms and both legs (not pictured), hold, then lower.

MODIFICATION

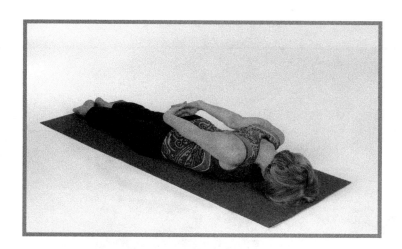

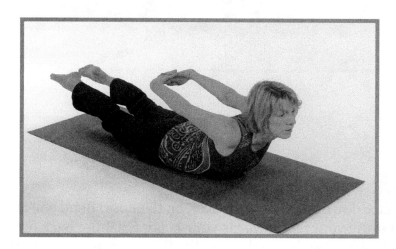

Variation 4: Bring your hands behind your back and interlock your fingers. On the inhale, raise your head, chest, and arms. Then raise your legs, hold, and breathe.

BOW

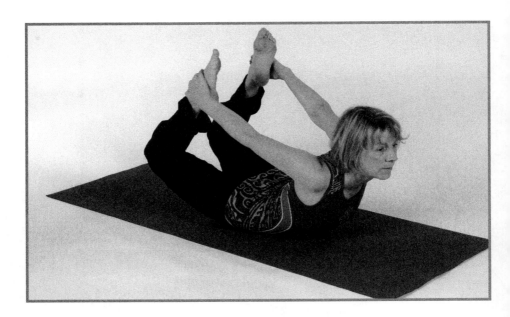

Lie face down with your forehead on the floor. Bend your knees and bring your feet towards your head, reaching back for your feet (a strap can be used to modify this pose, not pictured). On the inhale, raise your head and chest, then raise your legs, trying to bring your thighs off the floor. Work up to holding for five to six breaths, then repeat.

MODIFICATION

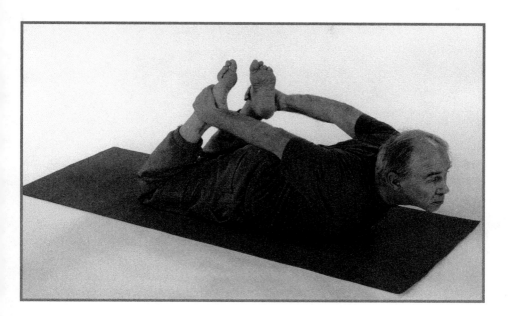

If you are unable to raise your thighs all the way, you can perform the poses as described, while keeping your thighs on the mat.

Note: As always, use caution and be sure to "listen" to your body—if the pose becomes too difficult, stop or switch to a more gentle variation.

UPWARD-FACING BENT LEG

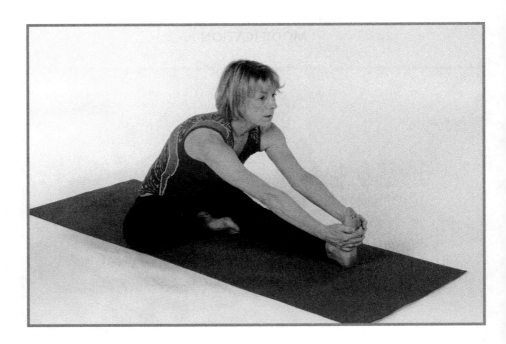

Sit tall and straight on the mat with both legs out in front of you, keeping your feet together. Bring your right leg in, placing the sole of your right foot against the inside of your left thigh. On the inhale, bring your arms overhead and look up at your hands. On the exhale, bend from your hips into a forward bend over your left leg, and reach as close to your foot as possible. Look at the horizon and hold for 5 breaths, then switch legs, and finish by performing the pose with both legs out (not pictured).

Note: As always, use caution and be sure to "listen" to your body—if the pose becomes too difficult, stop or switch to a more gentle variation.

CAT AND DOG

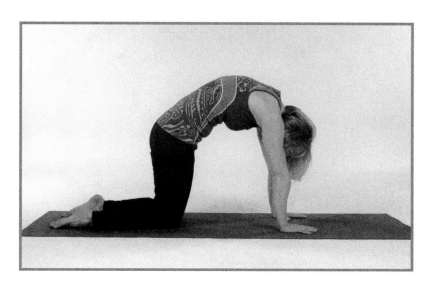

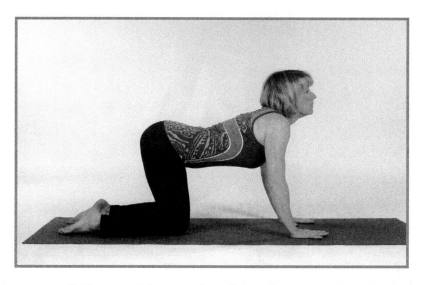

Start on all fours with your hands under your shoulders and your knees under your hips. On the exhale, round your back up to arch like a cat and bring your hips forward. Bring your chin to your chest. On the inhale, drop your belly and raise your head, pushing your sitting bones back and up. Repeat four to five times with the breath.

SIDE GATE

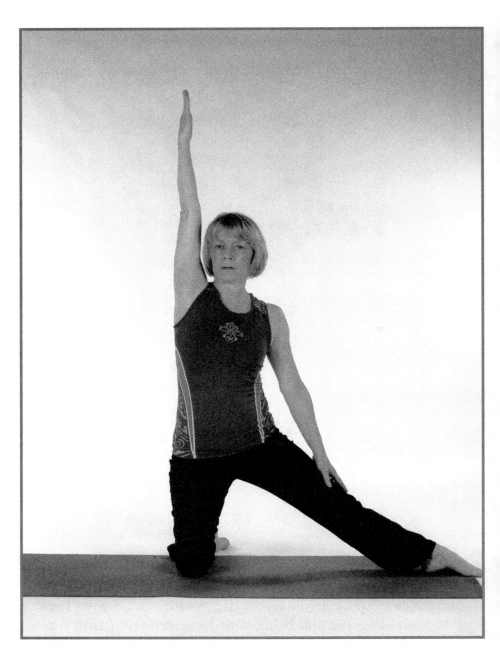

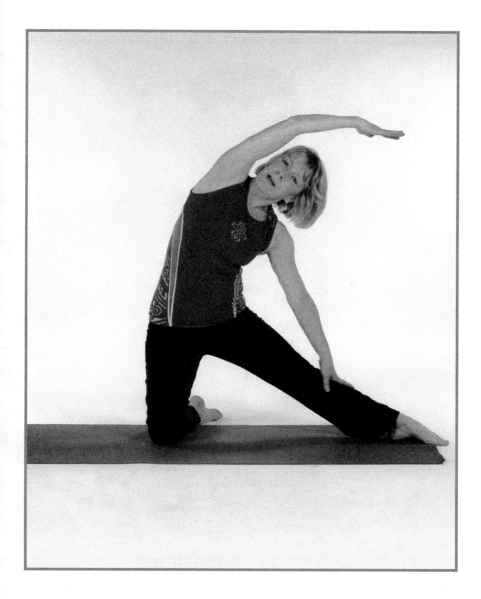

Come to your knees and extend your left leg straight out to the side. On the inhale, raise your right arm straight up. On the exhale, bend to the left, bringing your right arm over your head as your left arm moves down your leg. Hold for five breaths and repeat on the other side.

RABBIT

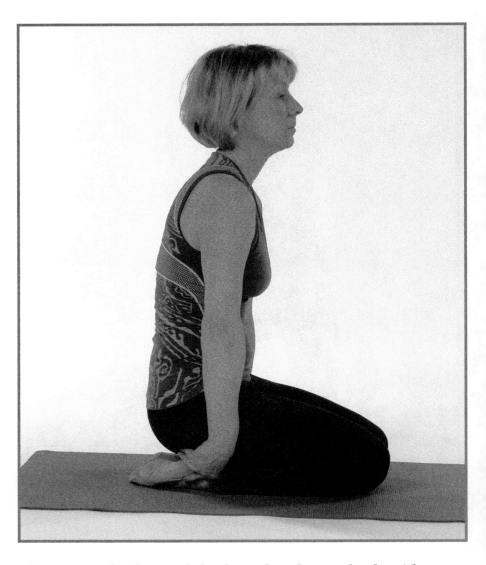

Sit on your heels, reach back, and grab your heels with your hands.

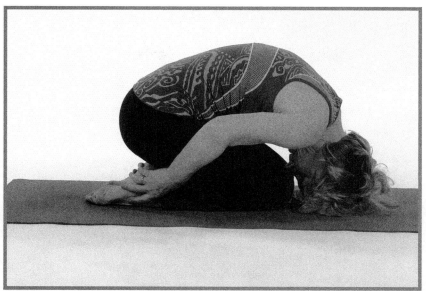

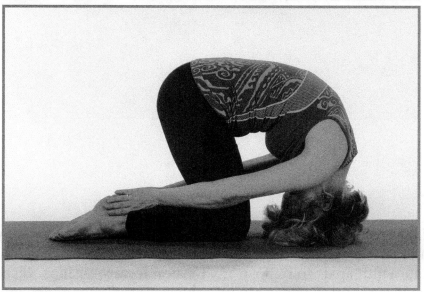

On the exhale, bend forward and bring your forehead as close as possible to your knees.

Raise your hips and roll to the top of your head (there will be a constriction in your throat). Hold and breathe slowly. Raise your head up and repeat once more.

CORPSE

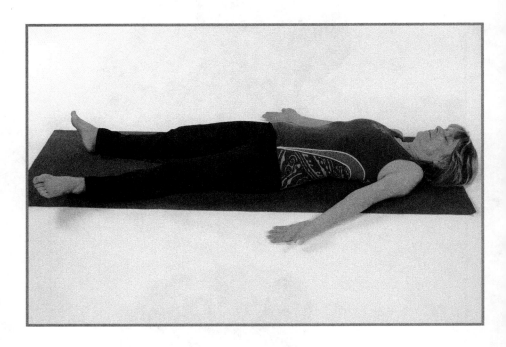

Lie on your back, with your arms extended out from your body and your palms facing up. Keep your legs a little more than hip-width apart to remove any tension from your hips. Close your eyes, bring your chin into the center of your chest, and keep your shoulders relaxed and away from your ears. Breathe deeply into your belly, letting your belly rise and fall with each breath. This pose is recommended at the end of your session to give your body a chance to relax and to allow the previous work from the poses to settle.

CHAPTER 5

GENTLE FLOWS FOR BACK PAIN

FLOOR BACK BENDS

POSE	PAGE	EQUIPMENT
Mountain	32	chair (optional)
Warm-Up Forward Bend	34	chair (optional)
Cat and Dog	79	
Sphinx	69	
Cobra	54	
Bow	76	
Reclined Spinal Twist	60	
Corpse	84	

STANDING CORE STRENGTHENING

POSE	PAGE	EQUIPMENT
Mountain	32	chair (optional)
Warm-Up Forward Bend	34	chair (optional)
Warrior II	38	chair (optional)
Reverse Warrior	42	chair (optional)
Lateral Stretch	48	
Reverse Triangle	46	block (optional)
Yoga Squat/Forward Bend	50	
Half Moon	44	block, chair (optional)
Corpse	84	

FLOOR CORE WORK

POSE	PAGE	EQUIPMENT
Mountain	32	chair (optional)
Warm-Up Forward Bend	34	chair (optional)
Bridge	62	
Fish	64	
Boat	66	chair (optional)
Side Gate	80	
Seated Twist	58	
Rabbit	82	
Corpse	84	

SPINAL TWIST

POSE	PAGE	EQUIPMENT
Mountain	32	chair (optional)
Warm-Up Forward Bend	34	chair (optional)
Reverse Triangle	46	block (optional)
Reclined Spinal Twist	60	
Recline Big Toe	70	strap (optional)
Seated Twist	58	
Upward-Facing Bent Leg	78	
Corpse	84	

BACK BENDS

POSE	PAGE	EQUIPMENT
Mountain	32	chair (optional)
Warm-Up Forward Bend	34	chair (optional)
Reverse Warrior	42	chair (optional)
Cat and Dog	79	
Bridge	62	
Cobra	54	
Bow	76	
Camel/Half Camel	56	block (optional)
Corpse	84	

REFERENCES

American Academy of Orthopaedic Surgeons
(AAOS)
www.aaos.org

American Chiropractic Association
www.acatoday.org

American Yoga Association
www.americanyogaassociation.org

International Association of Yoga Therapists
www.iayt.org

National Institute of Aging
www.nia.nih.gov

National Institute of Arthritis and Musculoskeletal
and Skin Diseases Information Clearinghouse
www.niams.nih.gov

National Institute of Neurological
Disorders and Stroke
www.ninds.nih.gov

North American Spine Society (NASS)
www.spine.org

Spine Health
www.spine-health.com

Yoga Journal
www.yogajournal.com

LAURIE SANFORD

Laurie Sanford has practiced yoga for 14 years and is certified under Rob Greenberg, owner of the Yoga for Peace Studio in Margaretville, NY. She has been teaching for eight years and currently provides yoga instruction to adults. Laurie has trained at the Kripalu Center for Yoga and Health, as well as the Himalayan Institute. She currently resides with her husband and daughter in the Catskill Mountains, where they run a weekly newspaper.

JO BRIELYN

Jo Brielyn is a freelance writer and author. She is a contributing writer for Hatherleigh Press and has published works in several print and online publications. Jo also owns and maintains the Creative Kids Ideas (www.creativekidsideas.com) and Good for Your Health (www.good-for-your-health.com) websites. For more information about Jo's upcoming projects or to contact her, visit www.JoBrielyn.com. Jo resides in Central Florida with her husband and two daughters.

Check Out These Other Titles from Hatherleigh Press!

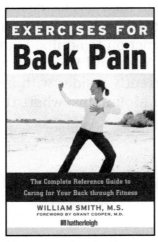

Exercises for Back Pain
ISBN 978-1-57826-304-2

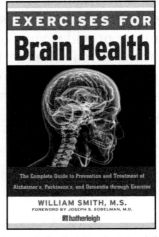

Exercises for Brain Health
ISBN 978-1-57826-316-5

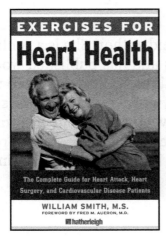

Exercises for Heart Health
ISBN 978-1-57826-303-5

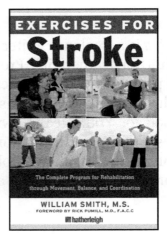

Exercises for Stroke
ISBN 978-1-57826-317-2

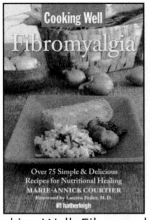
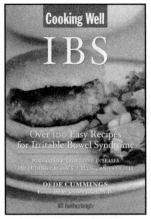

Cooking Well: Fibromyalgia
ISBN 978-1-57826-362-2

Cooking Well: IBS
ISBN 978-1-57826-388-2

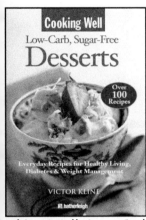
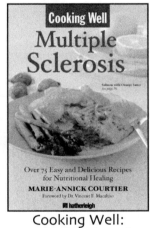
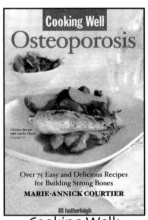

Cooking Well: Low-Carb
Sugar-Free Desserts
ISBN 978-1-57826-325-7

Cooking Well:
Multiple Sclerosis
ISBN 978-1-57826-301-1

Cooking Well:
Osteoporosis
ISBN 978-1-57826-302-8

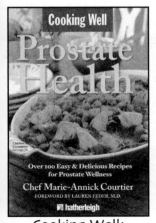
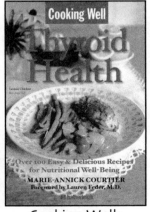
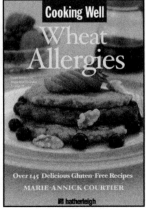

Cooking Well:
Prostate Health
ISBN 978-1-57826-376-9

Cooking Well:
Thyroid Health
ISBN 978-1-57826-352-3

Cooking Well:
Wheat Allergies
ISBN 978-1-57826-313-4